CONGESTIVE HEART FAILURE COOKBOOK FOR SENIORS

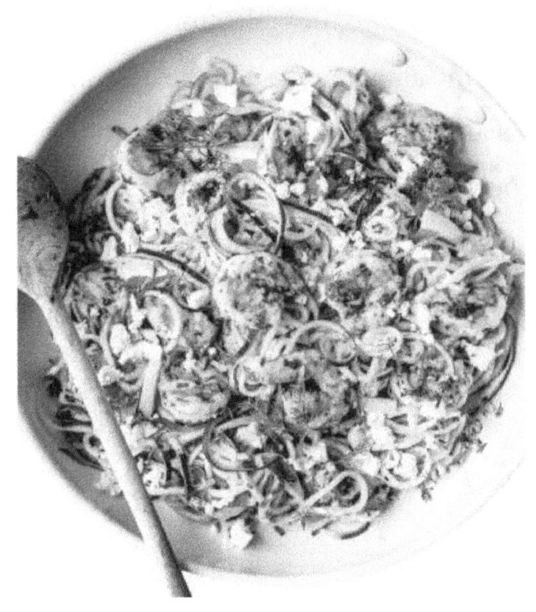

Delicious Dishes for Congestive Heart Failure Management

Linda Carlucci

Copyright © 2024 by Linda Carlucci

DISCLAIMER

This cookbook is intended to provide general information and recipes.

The recipes provided in this cookbook are not intended to replace or be a substitute for medical advice from a physician.

The reader should consult a healthcare professional for any specific medical advice, diagnosis or treatment.

Any specific dietary advice provided in this cookbook is not intended to replace or be a substitute for medical advice from a physician.

The author is not responsible or liable for any adverse effects experienced by readers of this cookbook as a result of following the recipes or dietary advice provided.

The author makes no representations or warranties of any kind (express or implied) as to the accuracy, completeness, reliability or suitability of the recipes provided in this cookbook.

The author disclaims any and all liability for any damages arising out of the use or misuse of the recipes provided in this cookbook. The reader must also take care to ensure that the recipes provided in this cookbook are prepared and cooked safely.

The recipes provided in this cookbook are for informational purposes only and should not be used as a substitute for professional medical advice, diagnosis or treatment.

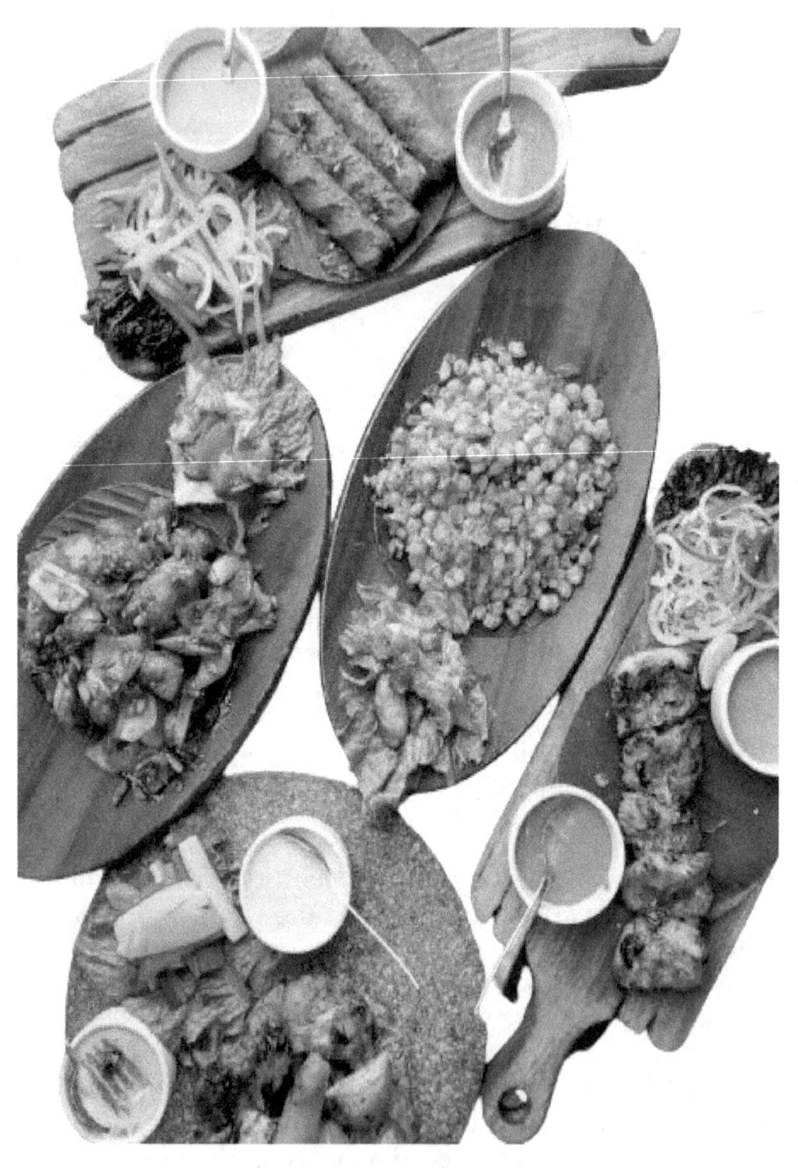

TABLE OF CONTENTS

INTRODUCTION

In the golden years of life, maintaining heart health becomes paramount, and understanding conditions like congestive heart failure (CHF) is crucial for seniors embarking on a journey to optimal well-being.

This book aims to unravel the complexities of CHF, providing insightful knowledge tailored to the unique needs of seniors.

Congestive heart failure refers to a condition where the heart struggles to pump blood effectively, leading to a gradual decline in its ability to meet the body's demands.

As you age, the risk of developing CHF increases, making it imperative for seniors to comprehend its intricacies. This book delves into the physiological aspects of CHF, demystifying medical jargon to empower seniors with a comprehensive understanding.

The negative impacts of congestive heart failure on seniors extend beyond the physical realm, affecting daily life and overall well-being. Fatigue, shortness of breath, and swelling in the legs can diminish one's quality of life, limiting the ability to engage in activities once enjoyed. Mental and emotional well-being can also be compromised as individuals grapple with the challenges posed by CHF.

As you navigate through the pages of this book, you will explore the far-reaching consequences of CHF, shedding light on the ways it can influence various aspects of your life.

Through knowledge, this book aims to help you to make informed decisions about your health, adopt preventive measures, and explore lifestyle modifications that can positively impact your heart health.

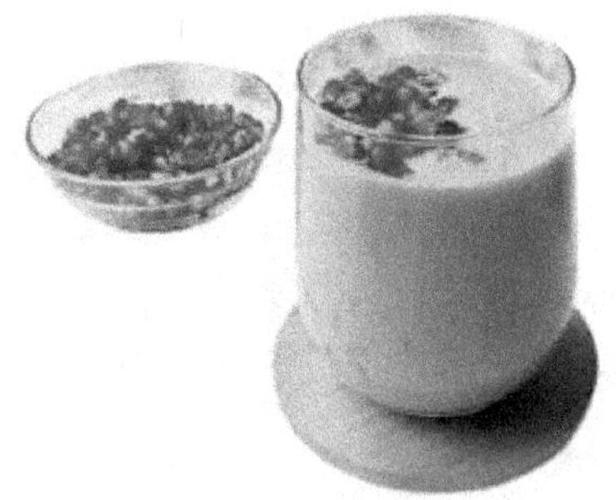

CHAPTER 1

BENEFITS OF A LOW CHOLESTEROL DIET FOR MANAGING CONGESTIVE HEART FAILURE

1. **Heart Health:** A low cholesterol diet helps maintain heart health by reducing the risk of atherosclerosis, which is crucial for managing congestive heart failure (CHF).

2. **Blood Pressure Control:** Lowering cholesterol intake supports better blood pressure management, a key factor in CHF care to reduce strain on the heart.

3. **Weight Management:** A low cholesterol diet aids in weight control, promoting overall cardiovascular well-being and easing the workload on the heart.

4. **Reduced Inflammation:** Lowering cholesterol intake can help minimize inflammation in blood vessels, contributing to improved heart function in CHF patients.

5. **Optimal Lipid Profile:** Maintaining a balanced lipid profile through a low cholesterol diet supports a

healthier cardiovascular system, vital for those with congestive heart failure.

6. **Improved Blood Flow:** By preventing cholesterol buildup in arteries, this diet ensures better blood flow, enhancing oxygen and nutrient delivery to the heart.

7. **Enhanced Exercise Tolerance**: A low cholesterol diet can improve exercise tolerance, assisting CHF patients in engaging in physical activities crucial for their well-being.

8. **Stabilized Blood Sugar Levels:** This diet can help stabilize blood sugar levels, contributing to better overall metabolic health for CHF patients.

9. **Reduced Risk of Clots:** Lowering cholesterol minimizes the risk of blood clots, which is essential in preventing complications related to congestive heart failure.

10. **Heart Rhythm Regulation:** A low cholesterol diet supports better regulation of heart rhythms, vital for managing CHF symptoms effectively.

11. **Antioxidant Benefits**: Foods rich in antioxidants, often part of a low cholesterol diet, can help protect

the heart from oxidative stress associated with congestive heart failure.

12. **Lowered Triglycerides:** This diet can contribute to reducing triglyceride levels, promoting a more favorable lipid profile for individuals with CHF.

13. **Improved Endothelial Function:** By supporting healthy endothelial function, a low cholesterol diet helps maintain the integrity of blood vessels, crucial for CHF patients.

14. **Lessened Fluid Retention:** Some components of a low cholesterol diet, such as potassium-rich foods, may help in managing fluid retention often seen in congestive heart failure.

15. **Overall Cardiovascular Support:** Adopting a low cholesterol diet provides comprehensive cardiovascular support, addressing multiple factors that are critical in the management of congestive heart failure.

DASH DIET AND IT'S BENEFIT FOR HEART HEALTH

1. **Fruits and Vegetables:** Rich in potassium, fiber, and antioxidants, they help lower blood pressure and reduce the risk of heart disease.

2. **Whole Grains:** Provide essential nutrients, fiber, and help regulate blood pressure and cholesterol levels.

3. **Lean Proteins**: Choose poultry, fish, beans, and nuts for protein without excessive saturated fat.

4. **Nuts and Seeds**: Contain healthy fats, fiber, and antioxidants, contributing to heart health.

5. **Low-Fat Dairy:** Good sources of calcium and protein with reduced saturated fat for overall cardiovascular support.

6. **Limit Red Meat:** Reducing red meat lowers saturated fat intake, promoting heart health.

7. **Healthy Fats:** Go for unsaturated fats found in olive oil, avocados, and fatty fish, supporting heart function.

8. **Low Sodium:** Reducing salt intake helps manage blood pressure, lowering the risk of heart disease.

9. **Limit Sweets:** Minimizing added sugars contributes to weight management and cardiovascular health.

10. **Portion Control:** Moderating portion sizes aids in maintaining a healthy weight and heart function.

11. **Moderate Alcohol:** If consumed, limit alcohol intake, as excessive alcohol can negatively impact heart health.

12. **Balanced Diet:** Combining various food groups ensures a diverse range of nutrients for overall heart well-being.

13. **Hydration:** Staying adequately hydrated supports overall health and cardiovascular function.

14. **Physical Activity:** Regular exercise complements the DASH diet, promoting heart health and overall well-being.

15. **Stress Management:** Incorporate stress-reducing activities like meditation or yoga, as chronic stress can impact heart health.

PRACTICAL WAYS TO REDUCE SODIUM IN YOUR DIET

1. **Read Labels**: Check food labels for sodium content and choose lower-sodium options.

2. **Fresh Produce:** Opt for fresh fruits and vegetables, as they are naturally low in sodium.

3. **Limit Processed Foods:** Processed foods often contain high sodium levels, so minimize their consumption.

4. **Cook at Home:** Prepare meals at home to have better control over ingredients and sodium levels.

5. **Use Herbs and Spices:** Enhance flavor with herbs, spices, and other seasonings instead of salt.

6. **Choose Low-Sodium Products:** Select products labeled as low-sodium or sodium-free when available.

7. **Rinse Canned Foods:** Rinse canned vegetables, beans, and fish to reduce sodium content.

8. **Limit Condiments:** Cut back on high-sodium condiments like soy sauce, ketchup, and pickles.

9. **Go Lean with Protein:** Choose lean protein sources like poultry, fish, and legumes over processed meats.

10. **Homemade Broths:** Make your own broths to control sodium levels in soups and stews.

11. **Educate Yourself:** Learn about hidden sources of sodium, such as baking soda and certain medications.

12. **Mindful Eating Out:** Be cautious when dining out and inquire about low-sodium options or adjustments.

13. **Portion Control:** Keep portions in check to manage overall sodium intake.

14. **Hydration:** Drink plenty of water to help flush out excess sodium from your system.

15. **Gradual Reduction:** Gradually reduce salt in recipes, allowing your taste buds to adjust over time.

SIMPLE EXERCISES FOR SENIORS WITH CONGESTIVE HEART FAILURE

1. **Walking:** A low-impact exercise that improves cardiovascular health and helps maintain mobility.

2. **Seated Leg Lifts:** While seated, lift one leg at a time to strengthen leg muscles and improve circulation.

3. **Arm Circles:** Rotate your arms in circular motions to enhance shoulder flexibility and strengthen arm muscles.
4. **Chair Squats:** Stand up from a seated position, using a chair for support, to engage leg muscles and improve balance.
5. **Marching in Place:** A simple way to elevate heart rate and promote circulation without high impact.
6. **Heel Raises:** Rise onto your toes to strengthen calf muscles and enhance lower leg circulation.
7. **Side Leg Raises:** While seated or standing, lift one leg to the side to engage hip muscles and improve stability.
8. **Deep Breathing:** Focus on slow, deep breaths to enhance lung capacity and reduce stress.
9. **Stationary Cycling:** Use a stationary bike for a low-impact cardiovascular workout that's gentle on the joints.
10. **Gentle Stretching:** Incorporate gentle stretches to improve flexibility and reduce muscle stiffness.

11. **Water Aerobics:** Perform exercises in a pool to reduce impact on joints while providing resistance for strength training.

12. **Seated Rowing:** Mimic rowing motions while seated to strengthen the back and arm muscles.

13. **Wall Push-Ups:** Perform push-ups against a wall to build upper body strength without strain.

14. **Balance Exercises:** Stand on one leg or use stability exercises to enhance balance and reduce the risk of falls.

15. **Tai Chi or Yoga:** These gentle, low-impact exercises promote flexibility, balance, and relaxation.

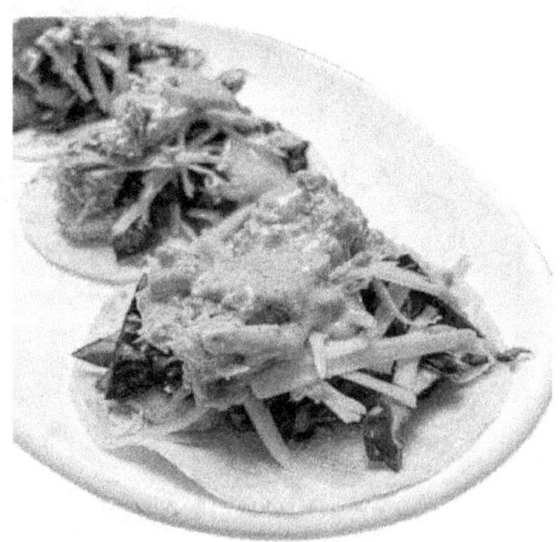

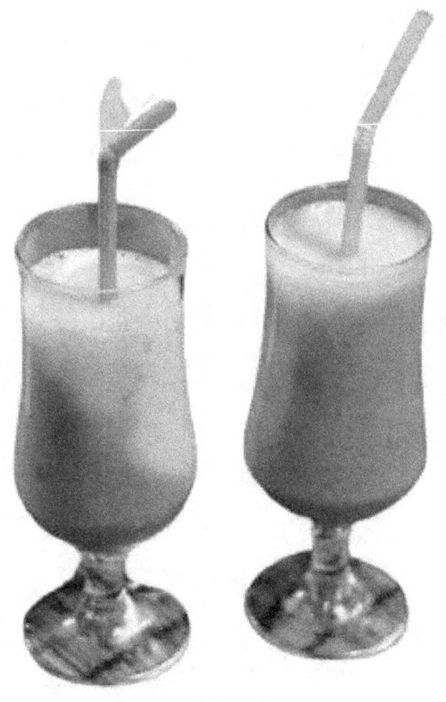

CHAPTER 2

14-DAY MEAL PLAN

DAY 1

Breakfast: Pistachio & Peach Toast

Lunch: Mediterranean Broccoli Pasta Salad

Dinner: Oven-Roasted Salmon with Charred Lemon Vinaigrette

DAY 2

Breakfast: Mango Raspberry Smoothie

Lunch: Mixed Greens with Lentils & Sliced Apple

Dinner: Chicken Kebabs

DAY 3

Breakfast: Spinach, Peanut Butter & Banana Smoothie

Lunch: Veggie & Hummus Sandwich

Dinner: Shrimp Scampi with Zoodles

DAY 4

Breakfast: Pineapple-Grapefruit Detox Smoothie:

Lunch: Peach & Spinach Salad with Feta

Dinner: Morning Burritos with Salsa Verde

DAY 5

Breakfast: Oatmeal with Berries and Low-Fat Milk

Lunch: Sichuan Ramen Cup of Noodles with Cabbage & Tofu

Dinner: Cauliflower Fried Rice

DAY 6

Breakfast: Breakfast Burrito

Lunch: Green Goddess Quinoa Bowls with Arugula & Shrimp

Dinner: Grilled Squash Garlic Bread

DAY 7

Breakfast: Pomegranate Smoothie

Lunch: Grilled Blackened Shrimp Tacos

Dinner: Pasta with Walnut Pesto and Peas

DAY 8

Breakfast: Overnight Oats

Lunch: Quinoa, Avocado & Chickpea Salad over Mixed Greens

Dinner: Chicken Salad Collard Wrap

DAY 9

Breakfast: Blueberry Lemon Oatmeal Parfaits

Lunch: Vegan Superfood Grain Bowls

Dinner: Butternut Squash and Turmeric Soup

DAY 10

Breakfast: Spinach Omelet Breakfast Sandwich

Lunch: Stuffed Sweet Potato with Hummus Dressing

Dinner: Baked Chicken Cutlets with Pineapple Rice

DAY 11

Breakfast: Pistachio & Peach Toast

Lunch: Mediterranean Broccoli Pasta Salad

Dinner: Oven-Roasted Salmon with Charred Lemon Vinaigrette

DAY 12

Breakfast: Mango Raspberry Smoothie

Lunch: Mixed Greens with Lentils & Sliced Apple

Dinner: Chicken Kebabs

DAY 13

Breakfast: Spinach, Peanut Butter & Banana Smoothie

Lunch: Veggie & Hummus Sandwich

Dinner: Shrimp Scampi with Zoodles

DAY 14

Breakfast: Pineapple-Grapefruit Detox Smoothie:

Lunch: Peach & Spinach Salad with Feta

Dinner: Morning Burritos with Salsa Verde

CHAPTER 3

NUTRITIOUS RECIPES CONGESTIVE HEART FAILURE DIET

BREAKFAST

Pistachio & Peach Toast

Preparation Time: 10 minutes

Serves: 2

Calories: 220 **Protein:** 7g **Fat:** 10g **Carbs:**29g
Cholesterol: 0m

Ingredients:

4 slices whole-grain, low-sodium bread

1 cup fresh peaches, sliced

1/2 cup unsalted pistachios, chopped

1 tablespoon honey (optional)

1 teaspoon cinnamon

Method of Preparation:

1. Toast the whole-grain bread slices.
2. Spread sliced peaches evenly over each slice.
3. Sprinkle chopped pistachios on top.
4. Drizzle with honey if desired.
5. Finish with a sprinkle of cinnamon.
6. Serving Information:

Mango Raspberry Smoothie

Preparation Time: 5 minutes

Serves: 2

Calories: 180 **Protein:** 8g **Fat:** 6g **Carbs:** 28g **Cholesterol:** 5mg

Ingredients:

1 cup frozen mango chunks

1/2 cup fresh raspberries

1 cup low-sodium almond milk

1/2 cup Greek yogurt (unsweetened)

1 tablespoon chia seeds

Method of Preparation:

1. Combine frozen mango, raspberries, almond milk, Greek yogurt, and chia seeds in a blender.
2. Blend until smooth.
3. Pour into glasses and serve.

Spinach, Peanut Butter & Banana Smoothie

Preparation Time: 5 minutes

Serves: 2

Calories: 250 **Protein:** 8g **Fat:** 14g **Carbs:** 27g
Cholesterol: 0mg

Ingredients:

2 cups fresh spinach

2 medium bananas, peeled

2 tablespoons natural peanut butter (unsalted)

1 cup unsweetened almond milk

1/2 teaspoon vanilla extract

Method of Preparation:

1. Place spinach, bananas, peanut butter, almond milk, and vanilla extract in a blender.
2. Blend until smooth.
3. Pour into glasses and serve.

Pineapple-Grapefruit Detox Smoothie

Preparation Time: 10 minutes

Serves: 2

Calories: 120 **Protein:** 2g **Fat:** 1g **Carbs:** 28g **Cholesterol:** 0mg

Ingredients:

1 cup fresh pineapple chunks

1 cup grapefruit segments

1/2 cup cucumber, peeled and sliced

1 tablespoon chia seeds

1 cup coconut water (unsweetened)

Ice cubes (optional)

Method of Preparation:

1. Combine pineapple, grapefruit, cucumber, chia seeds, and coconut water in a blender.
2. Blend until smooth.
3. Add ice cubes if desired and blend again.
4. Pour into glasses and serve immediately.

Oatmeal with Berries and Low-Fat Milk

Preparation Time: 15 minutes

Serves: 2

Calories: 280 **Protein:** 11g **Fat:** 5g **Carbs:** 48g **Cholesterol:** 10mg

Ingredients:

1 cup old-fashioned oats

2 cups low-fat milk

1 cup mixed berries (strawberries, blueberries, raspberries)

1 tablespoon honey (optional)

1/4 teaspoon cinnamon

Method of Preparation:

1. Cook oats in low-fat milk according to package instructions.
2. Once cooked, divide into two bowls.
3. Top each bowl with mixed berries, drizzle with honey if desired, and sprinkle with cinnamon.

Breakfast Burrito

Preparation Time: 20 minutes

Serves: 2

Calories: 320 **Protein:** 20g **Fat:** 8g **Carbs:** 40g **Cholesterol:** 30mg

Ingredients:

4 egg whites

1/2 cup black beans (canned, rinsed)

1/4 cup diced tomatoes

2 tablespoons diced onions

2 tablespoons chopped bell peppers

2 whole-grain tortillas

1/4 cup low-fat shredded cheese

Fresh cilantro (optional)

Method of Preparation:

1. In a non-stick pan, sauté onions and bell peppers until softened.
2. Add egg whites and scramble until fully cooked.
3. Warm tortillas in a dry pan or microwave.
4. Assemble burritos with scrambled eggs, black beans, tomatoes, and cheese.
5. Garnish with fresh cilantro if desired.

Pomegranate Smoothie

Preparation Time: 5 minutes

Serves:2

Calories: 180 **Protein:** 9g **Fat:** 5g **Carbs:** 28g
Cholesterol: 0mg

Ingredients:

1 cup pomegranate seeds (fresh or frozen)

1/2 cup low-fat Greek yogurt

1/2 cup almond milk (unsweetened)

1/2 banana

1 tablespoon chia seeds

1 teaspoon honey (optional)

Method of Preparation:

1. Combine pomegranate seeds, Greek yogurt, almond milk, banana, chia seeds, and honey in a blender.
2. Blend until smooth.
3. Pour into two glasses and serve chilled.

Overnight Oats

Preparation Time: 10 minutes

Serves: 2

Calories: 250 **Protein:** 8g **Fat:** 10g **Carbs:** 34g **Cholesterol:** 0mg

Ingredients:

1 cup rolled oats

1 cup almond milk (unsweetened)

1/2 cup fresh berries (blueberries or strawberries)

1 tablespoon chia seeds

1 tablespoon sliced almonds

1 teaspoon honey (optional)

Method of Preparation:

1. In a bowl, mix rolled oats, almond milk, chia seeds, and honey.
2. Divide the mixture into two jars.
3. Top each jar with fresh berries and sliced almonds.
4. Seal the jars and refrigerate overnight.
5. Serve chilled.

Blueberry Lemon Oatmeal Parfaits

Preparation Time: 15 minutes

Serves: 2

Calories: 280 **Protein:** 12g **Fat:** 8g **Carbs:** 42g
Cholesterol: 5mg

Ingredients:

1 cup cooked steel-cut oats

1/2 cup blueberries

1 tablespoon sliced almonds

1 teaspoon lemon zest

1/2 cup low-fat Greek yogurt

1 teaspoon honey (optional)

Method of Preparation:

1. In a glass or bowl, layer half of the cooked oats.
2. Add a layer of Greek yogurt, followed by blueberries and sliced almonds.
3. Repeat the layers.
4. Top with lemon zest and drizzle with honey.

Spinach Omelet Breakfast Sandwich

Preparation Time: 15 minutes

Serves: 2

Calories: 320 **Protein:** 22g **Fat:** 14g **Carbs:**25g
Cholesterol: 50mg

Ingredients:

4 large eggs

1 cup fresh spinach, chopped

1/4 cup red bell pepper, diced

2 whole grain English muffins

1 medium tomato, sliced

2 slices low-sodium turkey or chicken breast

1 tablespoon olive oil

Pepper

Method of Preparation:

1. In a bowl, whisk together eggs and add chopped spinach and diced red bell pepper.
2. Season with a pinch of salt and pepper.
3. Heat olive oil in a non-stick skillet over medium heat.
4. Pour the egg mixture into the skillet, allowing it to cook until the edges set.
5. Carefully flip the omelet and cook the other side until fully cooked.

6. Toast the English muffins and place each omelet on the bottom half.

7. Layer with sliced tomato and a slice of low-sodium turkey or chicken breast.

8. Top with the other half of the English muffin to create a sandwich.

Lunch

Mediterranean Broccoli Pasta Salad

Preparation Time: 25 minutes

Serves:2

Calories: 350 **Protein:** 10g **Fat:** 15g **Carbs:** 45g **Cholesterol:** 50mg

Ingredients:

1 cup whole wheat pasta

2 cups broccoli florets

1 cup cherry tomatoes, halved

1/2 cup black olives, sliced (low-sodium)

1/4 cup red onion, finely chopped

2 tablespoons extra-virgin olive oil

2 tablespoons balsamic vinegar

1 teaspoon dried oregano

Pepper

Method of Preparation:

1. Cook the whole wheat pasta according to package instructions.
2. Drain and let it cool.
3. Steam or blanch broccoli until tender-crisp.
4. Rinse under cold water and drain.
5. In a large bowl, combine pasta, broccoli, cherry tomatoes, olives, and red onion.
6. In a small bowl, whisk together olive oil, balsamic vinegar, dried oregano, salt, and pepper.
7. Pour the dressing over the pasta mixture and toss gently to combine.
8. Refrigerate for at least 30 minutes before serving.

Mixed Greens with Lentils & Sliced Apple

Preparation Time: 15 minutes

Serves: 2

Calories: 320 **Protein:** 12g **Fat:** 18g **Carbs:** 30g

Sodium: 600mg **Cholesterol:** 40mg

Ingredients:

4 cups mixed salad greens

1 cup cooked lentils

1 apple, thinly sliced

1/4 cup walnuts, chopped

2 tablespoons olive oil

1 tablespoon apple cider vinegar

1 teaspoon Dijon mustard

Pepper

Method of Preparation:

1. In a large bowl, combine mixed greens, cooked lentils, sliced apple, and chopped walnuts.
2. In a small bowl, whisk together olive oil, apple cider vinegar, Dijon mustard, salt, and pepper.
3. Drizzle the dressing over the salad and toss gently to coat.

Veggie & Hummus Sandwich

Preparation Time: 15 minutes

Serves: 2

Calories: 350 **Protein:** 12g **Fat:** 15g **Carbs:** 45g **Cholesterol:** 0mg

Ingredients:

4 slices whole-grain bread (low-sodium)

1 cup hummus (homemade or low-sodium store-bought)

1 cucumber, thinly sliced

1 large tomato, sliced

1 cup spinach leaves

1/2 red onion, thinly sliced

1 avocado, sliced

Ground black pepper to taste

Method of Preparation:

1. Spread hummus on each slice of bread.
2. Layer cucumber, tomato, spinach, red onion, and avocado evenly on two slices.
3. Sprinkle black pepper to taste.
4. Top with the remaining slices of bread to create two sandwiches.
5. Cut each sandwich in half.

Peach & Spinach Salad with Feta

Preparation Time: 10 minutes

Serves: 2

Calories: 280 **Protein:** 8g **Fat:** 20g **Carbs:** 20g **Cholesterol:** 20mg

Ingredients:

4 cups fresh spinach leaves

2 ripe peaches, sliced

1/2 cup crumbled feta cheese (low-sodium)

1/4 cup walnuts, chopped

2 tablespoons balsamic vinaigrette (low-sodium)

Method of Preparation:

1. In a large bowl, combine spinach, peach slices, feta, and walnuts.
2. Drizzle with balsamic vinaigrette and toss gently to coat.
3. Serve immediately.

Sichuan Ramen Cup of Noodles with Cabbage & Tofu

Preparation Time: 20 minutes

Serves: 2

Calories: 320 **Protein:** 15g **Fat:** 12g **Carbs:** 40g **Cholesterol:** 0mg

Ingredients:

2 cups cooked ramen noodles (low-sodium)

1 cup cabbage, shredded

1/2 cup firm tofu, cubed

1 tablespoon low-sodium soy sauce

1 teaspoon sesame oil

1/2 teaspoon Sichuan pepper (optional)

Green onions for garnish

Method of Preparation:

1. In a pan, sauté cabbage and tofu with soy sauce, sesame oil, and Sichuan pepper until tender.
2. Toss in cooked ramen noodles and mix well.
3. Garnish with green onions.

Green Goddess Quinoa Bowls with Arugula & Shrimp

Preparation Time: 25 minutes

Serves: 2

Calories: 520 **Protein:** 35g **Fat:** 24g **Carbs:** 42g
Cholesterol: 55mg

Ingredients:

1 cup quinoa, rinsed

1 ¾ cups low-sodium vegetable broth

1 lb. shrimp, peeled and deveined

2 cups arugula

1 avocado, sliced

½ cup cherry tomatoes, halved

¼ cup pumpkin seeds

2 tablespoons extra virgin olive oil

2 tablespoons lemon juice

1 clove garlic, minced

Pepper

Fresh parsley for garnish (optional)

Method of Preparation:

1. In a saucepan, combine quinoa and vegetable broth. Bring to a boil, then reduce heat, cover, and simmer for 15 minutes or until quinoa is cooked.

2. Season shrimp with black pepper and grill for 2-3 minutes on each side until opaque.

3. In a large bowl, combine cooked quinoa, arugula, avocado slices, cherry tomatoes, and pumpkin seeds.

4. Whisk together olive oil, lemon juice, minced garlic, salt, and pepper.

5. Drizzle over the quinoa mixture and toss gently.

6. Divide the quinoa mixture into two bowls, top with grilled shrimp, and garnish with fresh parsley if desired.

Grilled Blackened Shrimp Tacos

Preparation Time: 20 minutes

Serves: 2

Calories: 420 **Protein:** 28g **Fat:** 18g **Carbs:** 36g **Cholesterol:** 50mg

Ingredients:

1 lb. shrimp, peeled and deveined

1 tablespoon olive oil

1 teaspoon paprika

1 teaspoon garlic powder

1 teaspoon onion powder

1 teaspoon cumin

½ teaspoon cayenne pepper

¼ teaspoon black pepper

4 whole wheat tortillas

1 cup shredded cabbage

1 avocado, sliced

½ cup Greek yogurt (unsweetened)

Fresh cilantro for garnish

Method of Preparation:

1. In a bowl, mix olive oil, paprika, garlic powder, onion powder, cumin, cayenne pepper, and black pepper. Toss shrimp in the mixture until coated.
2. Grill shrimp for 2-3 minutes on each side until blackened and cooked through.
3. Warm tortillas on the grill or in a pan.

4. Assemble tacos by placing grilled shrimp on tortillas, topping with shredded cabbage, avocado slices, and a dollop of Greek yogurt.

5. Garnish with fresh cilantro.

Quinoa, Avocado & Chickpea Salad over Mixed Greens

Preparation Time: 20 minutes

Serves: 2

Calories: 420 **Protein:** 12g **Fat:** 22g **Carbs:** 47g **Cholesterol:** 0mg

Ingredients:

1 cup quinoa, rinsed

1 can (15 oz) low-sodium chickpeas, drained and rinsed

1 ripe avocado, diced

4 cups mixed greens (spinach, kale, arugula)

1 cup cherry tomatoes, halved

1/4 cup red onion, finely chopped

2 tablespoons extra-virgin olive oil

2 tablespoons balsamic vinegar

1 teaspoon Dijon mustard

Pepper

Method of Preparation:

1. Cook quinoa according to package instructions.
2. Let it cool.
3. In a large bowl, combine quinoa, chickpeas, avocado, mixed greens, cherry tomatoes, and red onion.
4. In a small bowl, whisk together olive oil, balsamic vinegar, Dijon mustard, salt, and pepper to create the dressing.
5. Drizzle the dressing over the salad and toss gently to combine.

Vegan Superfood Grain Bowls

Preparation Time: 30 minutes

Serves: 2

Calories: 480 **Protein:** 18g **Fat:** 18g **Carbs:** 64g
Cholesterol: 0mg

Ingredients:

1 cup quinoa, rinsed

1 cup sweet potatoes, cubed

1 cup broccoli florets

1 cup kale, chopped

1 cup cooked black beans, drained

1/4 cup pumpkin seeds

2 tablespoons tahini

1 tablespoon lemon juice

1 clove garlic, minced

1 teaspoon cumin

Pepper

Method of Preparation:

1. Cook quinoa according to package instructions.

2. Roast sweet potatoes and broccoli in the oven at 400°F (200°C) for 20 minutes.

3. In a large bowl, assemble quinoa, roasted sweet potatoes, broccoli, kale, black beans, and pumpkin seeds.

4. In a small bowl, mix tahini, lemon juice, minced garlic, cumin, salt, and pepper to create the dressing.

5. Drizzle the dressing over the bowl and toss gently.

6. Divide into 2 servings.

Stuffed Sweet Potato with Hummus Dressing

Preparation Time: 15 minutes

Serves:2

Calories: 320 **Protein:** 8g **Fat:** 14g **Carbs:**42g
Cholesterol: 30mg

Ingredients:

2 medium sweet potatoes

1 cup canned chickpeas, drained and rinsed (low-sodium)

2 tablespoons tahini

2 tablespoons lemon juice

1 garlic clove, minced

1 tablespoon olive oil

1/2 teaspoon ground cumin

Salt substitute to taste

Freshly ground black pepper to taste

1/4 cup chopped fresh parsley (for garnish)

Method of Preparation:

1. Preheat the oven to 400°F (200°C).
2. Wash and pierce sweet potatoes with a fork. Bake for 45-60 minutes until tender.
3. In a food processor, combine chickpeas, tahini, lemon juice, minced garlic, olive oil, cumin, salt substitute, and black pepper.
4. Blend until smooth.
5. Once sweet potatoes are done, cut them in half and fluff the insides with a fork.
6. Stuff each sweet potato with the hummus dressing.
7. Garnish with chopped parsley.

Dinner

Oven-Roasted Salmon with Charred Lemon Vinaigrette

Preparation Time: 25 minutes

Serves: 2

Calories: 320 **Protein:** 24g **Fat:** 22g **Carbs:** 8g
Cholesterol: 45mg

Ingredients:

2 salmon fillets

1 tablespoon olive oil

1 teaspoon dried thyme

1 teaspoon garlic powder

Pepper

2 lemons (1 for roasting, 1 for vinaigrette)

2 tablespoons fresh parsley, chopped

Vinaigrette:

2 tablespoons olive oil

1 tablespoon Dijon mustard

1 teaspoon honey

1 clove garlic, minced

Method of Preparation:

1. Preheat the oven to 400°F (200°C).
2. Place salmon fillets on a baking sheet, drizzle with olive oil, and season with thyme, garlic powder, and pepper.
3. Roast salmon for 15-20 minutes or until cooked through.
4. While salmon cooks, cut one lemon in half. Place the halves, cut side down, in a hot, dry pan until charred.
5. For the vinaigrette, whisk together olive oil, Dijon mustard, honey, minced garlic, and the juice from the charred lemon.
6. Once salmon is done, drizzle with the vinaigrette, squeeze fresh lemon juice, and garnish with chopped parsley.

Chicken Kebabs

Preparation Time: 45 minutes

Serves: 2

Calories: 280 **Protein:** 32g **Fat:** 14g **Carbs:** 8g
Cholesterol: 50mg

Ingredients:

2 boneless, skinless chicken breasts, cut into cubes

1 tablespoon olive oil

1 teaspoon dried oregano

1 teaspoon paprika

Pepper

1 bell pepper, cut into chunks

1 zucchini, sliced

Marinade:

2 tablespoons low-sodium soy sauce

1 tablespoon olive oil

1 clove garlic, minced

1 teaspoon lemon juice

Method of Preparation:

1. In a bowl, combine chicken cubes, olive oil, oregano, paprika, salt, and pepper.
2. Allow it to marinate for at least 30 minutes.
3. Preheat grill or grill pan.
4. Thread marinated chicken, bell pepper, and zucchini onto skewers.
5. Grill kebabs for 12-15 minutes, turning occasionally, until chicken is fully cooked.

Shrimp Scampi with Zoodles

Preparation Time: 20 minutes

Serves: 2

Calories: 250 **Protein:** 28g **Fat:** 12g **Carbs:** 12g **Cholesterol:** 50mg

Ingredients:

1 Pound large shrimp, peeled and deveined

2 tablespoons olive oil

3 cloves garlic, minced

1/4 teaspoon red pepper flakes (optional)

Zest and juice of 1 lemon

4 medium zucchinis, spiralized into zoodles

2 tablespoons fresh parsley, chopped

Method of Preparation:

1. In a skillet, heat olive oil over medium heat.
2. Add minced garlic and red pepper flakes, sauté for 1-2 minutes.
3. Add shrimp, cook for 2-3 minutes per side until pink and opaque.
4. Add lemon zest and juice, then toss in the zoodles.
5. Cook for an additional 2-3 minutes until zoodles are tender.
6. Garnish with chopped parsley before serving.

Morning Burritos with Salsa Verde

Preparation Time: 20 minutes

Serves: 2

Calories: 480 **Protein:** 20g **Fat:** 22g **Carbs:** 52g
Cholesterol: 50mg

Ingredients:

4 whole wheat tortillas

4 large eggs, beaten

1 cup black beans, cooked and drained (low-sodium)

1 cup cherry tomatoes, diced

1/2 cup low-fat shredded cheddar cheese

1 avocado, sliced

1/4 cup fresh cilantro, chopped

Salsa Verde (low-sodium) for serving

Method of Preparation:

1. In a non-stick skillet, scramble the eggs until cooked through.
2. Warm the tortillas in a dry skillet or microwave.
3. Assemble the burritos by layering eggs, black beans, cherry tomatoes, cheese, avocado, and cilantro.

4. Roll the burritos and serve with a side of low-sodium Salsa Verde.

Cauliflower Fried Rice

Preparation Time: 25 minutes

Serves:2

Calories: 320 **Protein:** 28g **Fat:** 12g **Carbs:** 22g **Cholesterol:** 50mg

Ingredients:

4 cups cauliflower rice

1 cup cooked chicken breast, diced (low-sodium)

1 cup mixed vegetables (peas, carrots, corn), frozen

2 eggs, beaten

1 tablespoon sesame oil

1/2 cup green onions, chopped

Method of Preparation:

1. In a large skillet, sauté cauliflower rice, cooked chicken, and mixed vegetables until heated through.

2. Push the mixture to one side and scramble the eggs on the empty side.

3. Combine eggs with the rice mixture.

4. Add sesame oil, and green onions.

5. Stir well before serving.

Grilled Squash Garlic Bread

Preparation Time: 15 minutes

Serves: 2

Calories: 280 **Protein:** 8g **Fat:** 14g **Carbs:** 30g
Cholesterol: 0mg

Ingredients:

1 medium zucchini, sliced

1 medium yellow squash, sliced

4 slices whole-grain bread (low-sodium)

2 cloves garlic, minced

2 tablespoons olive oil

1 tablespoon fresh basil, chopped

Pepper

Method of Preparation:

1. Preheat grill or grill pan.

2. Brush zucchini and yellow squash with olive oil, sprinkle with salt and pepper.

3. Grill the squash slices until tender, about 3-4 minutes per side.

4. Toast the bread slices and rub with minced garlic.

5. Arrange grilled squash on top of the garlic-rubbed bread slices.

6. Drizzle with extra olive oil and sprinkle with fresh basil.

Pasta with Walnut Pesto and Peas

Preparation Time: 20 minutes

Serves: 2

Calories: 450 **Protein:** 15g **Fat:** 24g **Carbs: Cholesterol:** 25mg

Ingredients:

8 oz whole wheat pasta

1 cup frozen peas

1/2 cup walnuts, chopped

2 cups fresh basil leaves

1/4 cup extra virgin olive oil

1/4 cup Parmesan cheese, grated (low-sodium)

Pepper

Method of Preparation:

1. Cook pasta according to package instructions, adding peas in the last 3 minutes of cooking.
2. Drain and set aside.
3. In a food processor, combine walnuts, basil and Parmesan.
4. Pulse until finely chopped.
5. With the processor running, slowly add olive oil until a smooth pesto forms.
6. Season with pepper.
7. Toss the cooked pasta and peas with the walnut pesto.

Chicken Salad Collard Wrap

Preparation Time: 15 minutes

Serves: 2

Calories: 280 **Protein:** 30g **Fat:** 8g **Carbs:** 22g
Cholesterol: 40mg

Ingredients:

1 cup cooked chicken breast, shredded

1/2 cup celery, diced

1/4 cup red onion, finely chopped

1/4 cup low-fat Greek yogurt

1 tablespoon Dijon mustard

2 tablespoons fresh parsley, chopped

Pepper

4 large collard green leaves

Method of Preparation:

1. In a bowl, combine shredded chicken, celery, red onion, Greek yogurt, Dijon mustard, and parsley. Mix well.
2. Season with Pepper.
3. Steam collard green leaves for 1-2 minutes until pliable.

4. Spoon chicken salad into each collard leaf and wrap tightly.

Butternut Squash and Turmeric Soup

Preparation Time: 30 minutes

Serves: 2

Calories: 220 **Protein:** 4g **Fat:** 5g **Carbs:** 45g **Cholesterol:** 0mg

Ingredients:

1 medium butternut squash, peeled and diced

1 onion, chopped

2 carrots, peeled and sliced

1 teaspoon turmeric

4 cups low-sodium vegetable broth

1 tablespoon olive oil

Pepper

1/4 cup low-fat plain yogurt (optional, for garnish)

Method of Preparation:

1. In a large pot, heat olive oil and sauté onions until translucent.
2. Add butternut squash, carrots, turmeric, salt, and pepper. Cook for 5 minutes.
3. Pour in vegetable broth, bring to a boil, then reduce heat and simmer until vegetables are tender.
4. Use an immersion blender to puree the soup until smooth.
5. Serve hot, optionally garnished with a dollop of low-fat plain yogurt.

Baked Chicken Cutlets with Pineapple Rice

Preparation Time: 35 minutes

Serves: 2

Calories: 420 **Protein:** 30g **Fat:** 10g **Carbs:** 55g **Cholesterol:** 35mg

Ingredients:

2 boneless, skinless chicken breasts

1 cup brown rice, cooked

1 cup pineapple chunks (fresh or canned in juice), drained

1 tablespoon low-sodium soy sauce

1 tablespoon olive oil

1 teaspoon ginger, grated

1/2 teaspoon garlic powder

Pepper

Method of Preparation:

1. Preheat oven to 400°F (200°C).
2. Season chicken breasts with soy sauce, ginger, garlic powder, salt, and pepper.
3. Bake for 20-25 minutes until cooked through.
4. In a pan, sauté cooked rice with olive oil and pineapple chunks until heated through.
5. Slice baked chicken and serve over pineapple rice.

SEAFOOD MAINS

Pasta with Walnut Pesto and Peas

Preparation Time: 20 minutes

Serves: 2

Calories: 450 **Protein:** 15g **Fat:** 25g **Carbs:** 45g
Cholesterol: 30mg

Ingredients:

200g whole wheat pasta

1 cup frozen peas

1 cup fresh basil leaves

1/2 cup walnuts (unsalted)

1/4 cup olive oil

1/4 cup grated Parmesan cheese (low-sodium)

Pepper

Method of Preparation:

1. Cook pasta according to package instructions.
2. Add frozen peas during the last 2 minutes of boiling.
3. Drain and set aside.
4. In a food processor, blend basil, walnuts, and Parmesan.

5. Slowly add olive oil until a pesto consistency is achieved.

6. Season with pepper.

7. Toss the pasta and peas with the walnut pesto until well coated.

Lemon-Garlic Salmon Bites

Preparation Time: 25 minutes

Serves: 2

Calories: 320 **Protein:** 30g **Fat:** 20g **Carbs:** 2g **Cholesterol:** 50mg

Ingredients:

2 salmon fillets (about 150g each)

2 tablespoons olive oil

2 cloves garlic, minced

1 lemon (juiced and zested)

1 teaspoon dried oregano

Pepper

Fresh parsley for garnish (optional)

Method of Preparation:

1. Preheat oven to 375°F (190°C).

2. Place salmon fillets on a baking sheet lined with parchment paper.

3. In a bowl, mix olive oil, minced garlic, lemon juice, lemon zest, oregano, salt, and pepper.

4. Brush the mixture over the salmon.

5. Bake for 15-20 minutes or until salmon is cooked through.

6. Garnish with fresh parsley if desired.

Salmon Tikka Parcels with Rice Salad

Preparation Time: 30 minutes

Serves: 2

Calories: 480 **Protein:** 35g **Fat:** 15g **Carbs:** 45g **Cholesterol:** 40mg

Ingredients:

2 salmon fillets (about 150g each)

1 cup brown rice (cooked)

1 cup cucumber, diced

1 cup cherry tomatoes, halved

1/4 cup plain Greek yogurt (low-fat)

1 tablespoon tikka masala spice blend

1 tablespoon olive oil

Fresh cilantro for garnish (optional)

Method of Preparation:

1. Preheat oven to 375°F (190°C).
2. Place each salmon fillet on a piece of parchment paper.
3. Mix tikka masala spice with olive oil and rub it onto each salmon fillet.
4. Seal the parchment paper parcels and bake for 20 minutes.
5. In a bowl, mix cooked brown rice, cucumber, cherry tomatoes, and yogurt to create the rice salad.
6. Serve salmon parcels over a bed of rice salad.
7. Garnish with fresh cilantro if desired.

Seafood Chowder

Preparation Time: 35 minutes

Serves: 2

Calories: 400 **Protein:** 35g **Fat:** 12g **Carbs:** 40g
Cholesterol: 50mg

Ingredients:

1 cup shrimp, peeled and deveined

1 cup white fish fillets, diced

1 cup scallops

1 cup potatoes, diced

1 cup celery, chopped

1 cup carrots, sliced

1/2 cup leeks, sliced

3 cups low-sodium vegetable broth

1 cup low-fat milk

2 tablespoons olive oil

1 teaspoon dried thyme

Pepper

Method of Preparation:

1. In a large pot, sauté leeks, celery, and carrots in olive oil until softened.
2. Add potatoes, thyme, salt, and pepper.
3. Cook for another 5 minutes.
4. Pour in vegetable broth and bring to a simmer.
5. Add shrimp, fish, and scallops.
6. Cook until seafood is opaque and cooked through.
7. Stir in milk and heat until chowder is warmed through.

Fish with Moroccan Lentil Salad

Preparation Time: 30 minutes

Serves:2

Calories: 350 **Protein:** 30g **Fat:** 12g **Carbs:** 30g
Cholesterol: 50mg

Ingredients:

2 white fish fillets (e.g., tilapia or cod)

1 cup dried green or brown lentils, rinsed

1 cup cherry tomatoes, halved

1 cucumber, diced

1/4 cup red onion, finely chopped

2 tablespoons fresh parsley, chopped

2 tablespoons olive oil

1 teaspoon ground cumin

1 teaspoon ground coriander

1/2 teaspoon paprika

1/4 teaspoon cinnamon

Pepper

Method of Preparation:

1. Cook lentils according to package instructions; drain and set aside.
2. In a large bowl, combine cooked lentils, cherry tomatoes, cucumber, red onion, and parsley.

3. In a small bowl, mix olive oil, cumin, coriander, paprika, cinnamon, salt, and pepper to create the dressing.
4. Season fish fillets with salt and pepper, then bake or grill until cooked through.
5. Serve fish on a bed of Moroccan lentil salad, drizzle with dressing.

Italian Fish Parcels

Preparation Time: 25 minutes

Serves: 2

Calories: 320 **Protein:** 28g **Fat:** 16g **Carbs:** 18g **Cholesterol:** 50mg

Ingredients:

2 white fish fillets (e.g., haddock or sole)

1 cup cherry tomatoes, halved

1 zucchini, thinly sliced

2 tablespoons fresh basil, chopped

2 tablespoons olive oil

1 tablespoon lemon juice

1 teaspoon dried oregano

Pepper

Method of Preparation:

1. Preheat the oven to 375°F (190°C).
2. In a bowl, combine cherry tomatoes, zucchini, garlic, basil, olive oil, lemon juice, oregano, and pepper.
3. Cut two large squares of parchment paper. Place a fish fillet on each square.
4. Spoon vegetable mixture over each fish fillet.
5. Fold the parchment paper over the fish and vegetables, sealing the edges to create parcels.
6. Bake in the preheated oven for about 15-20 minutes or until the fish is cooked through.

POULTRY MAINS

Ham & Cheese Stuffed Chicken Breasts

Preparation Time: 40 minutes

Serves:2 **Calories:**   320 **Protein:** 45g **Fat:** 12g **Carbs:**2g **Sodium:** 800mg **Cholesterol:** 50mg

Ingredients:

2 boneless, skinless chicken breasts

2 slices low-sodium ham

2 slices low-sodium Swiss cheese

1 teaspoon olive oil

1/2 teaspoon black pepper

1/2 teaspoon dried thyme

1/2 teaspoon paprika

Fresh parsley for garnish (optional)

Method of Preparation:

1. Preheat oven to 375°F (190°C).
2. Make a horizontal slit in each chicken breast to form a pocket.
3. Stuff each pocket with a slice of ham and a slice of Swiss cheese.

4. Rub the chicken breasts with olive oil and season with black pepper, thyme, and paprika.

5. Place the chicken breasts in a baking dish and bake for 25-30 minutes or until the internal temperature reaches 165°F (74°C).

6. Garnish with fresh parsley if desired.

Easy Chicken Enchiladas

Preparation Time: 45 minutes

Serves:2

Calories: 480 **Protein:** 35g **Fat:** 14g **Carbs:**55g **Cholesterol:** 55mg

Ingredients:

2 boneless, skinless chicken breasts, cooked and shredded

4 whole wheat tortillas

1 cup low-sodium black beans, drained and rinsed

1 cup low-sodium corn kernels

1 cup diced tomatoes

1 cup shredded low-fat cheddar cheese

1 teaspoon chili powder

1/2 teaspoon cumin

1/2 teaspoon garlic powder

1/4 teaspoon black pepper

1 cup low-sodium enchilada sauce

Method of Preparation:

1. Preheat oven to 375°F (190°C).
2. In a bowl, combine shredded chicken, black beans, corn, diced tomatoes, 1/2 cup cheddar cheese, chili powder, cumin, and black pepper.
3. Fill each tortilla with the chicken mixture, roll, and place seam side down in a baking dish.
4. Pour enchilada sauce over the rolled tortillas and sprinkle the remaining 1/2 cup cheddar cheese on top.
5. Bake for 20-25 minutes or until cheese is melted and bubbly.

Spicy Chicken Tacos

Preparation Time: 40 minutes

Serves: 2

Calories: 380 **Protein:** 28g **Fat:** 12g **Carbs:** 38g
Cholesterol: 50mg

Ingredients:

1 lb. boneless, skinless chicken thighs

1 tsp smoked paprika

1 tsp cumin

1/2 tsp chili powder

1/4 tsp onion powder

1/4 tsp black pepper

1/4 tsp cayenne pepper

8 small whole wheat tortillas

1 cup shredded lettuce

1 cup diced tomatoes

1/2 cup diced onions

2 tbsp chopped fresh cilantro

1 lime (cut into wedges)

Method of Preparation:

1. Preheat oven to 375°F (190°C).
2. In a bowl, mix smoked paprika, cumin, chili powder, onion powder, black pepper, and cayenne pepper.
3. Rub the spice mixture over chicken thighs.
4. Bake chicken for 25-30 minutes or until fully cooked.
5. Shred the cooked chicken and assemble tacos with whole wheat tortillas, lettuce, tomatoes, onions, cilantro, and a squeeze of lime.

Chicken Thighs with Couscous & Kale

Preparation Time: 30 minutes

Serves: 2

Calories: 480 **Protein:** 35g **Fat:** 14g **Carbs:** 45g **Cholesterol:** 50mg

Ingredients:

1 lb. boneless, skinless chicken thighs

1 cup whole wheat couscous

2 cups chopped kale

1 tbsp olive oil

1 tsp garlic powder

1 tsp dried thyme

Pepper

Lemon wedges for serving

Method of Preparation:

1. Season chicken thighs with garlic powder, dried thyme, and pepper.
2. In a skillet, heat olive oil over medium-high heat. Cook chicken thighs until browned on both sides.
3. Cook whole wheat couscous according to package instructions.
4. In the same skillet, add chopped kale and cook until wilted.
5. Serve chicken over couscous and kale, with a squeeze of lemon.

Creamy Pesto Chicken Salad with Greens

Preparation Time: 25 minutes

Serves: 2

Calories: 320 **Protein:** 30g **Fat:** 15g **Carbs:** 18g **Cholesterol:** 50mg

Ingredients:

1 lb. boneless, skinless chicken breasts

2 cups mixed salad greens

1/4 cup low-sodium pesto

2 tbsp plain Greek yogurt

1 tbsp lemon juice

1 tsp Dijon mustard

Pepper

Cherry tomatoes for garnish

Method of Preparation:

1. Grill or bake chicken breasts until fully cooked.

2. In a bowl, mix low-sodium pesto, Greek yogurt, lemon juice, Dijon mustard, salt, and pepper to create the dressing.

3. Slice the cooked chicken and toss it with salad greens.

4. Drizzle the creamy pesto dressing over the salad and garnish with cherry tomatoes.

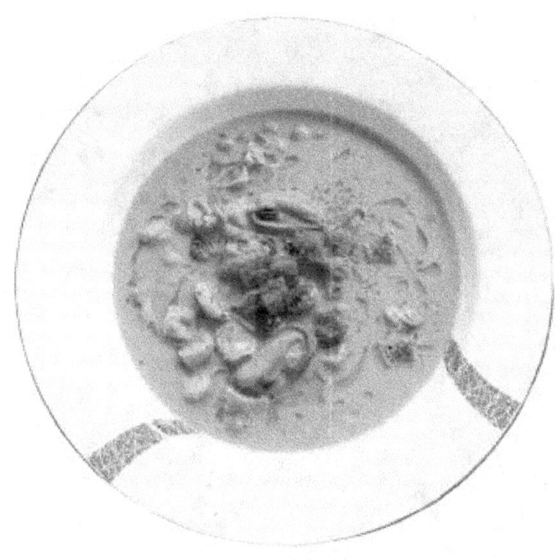

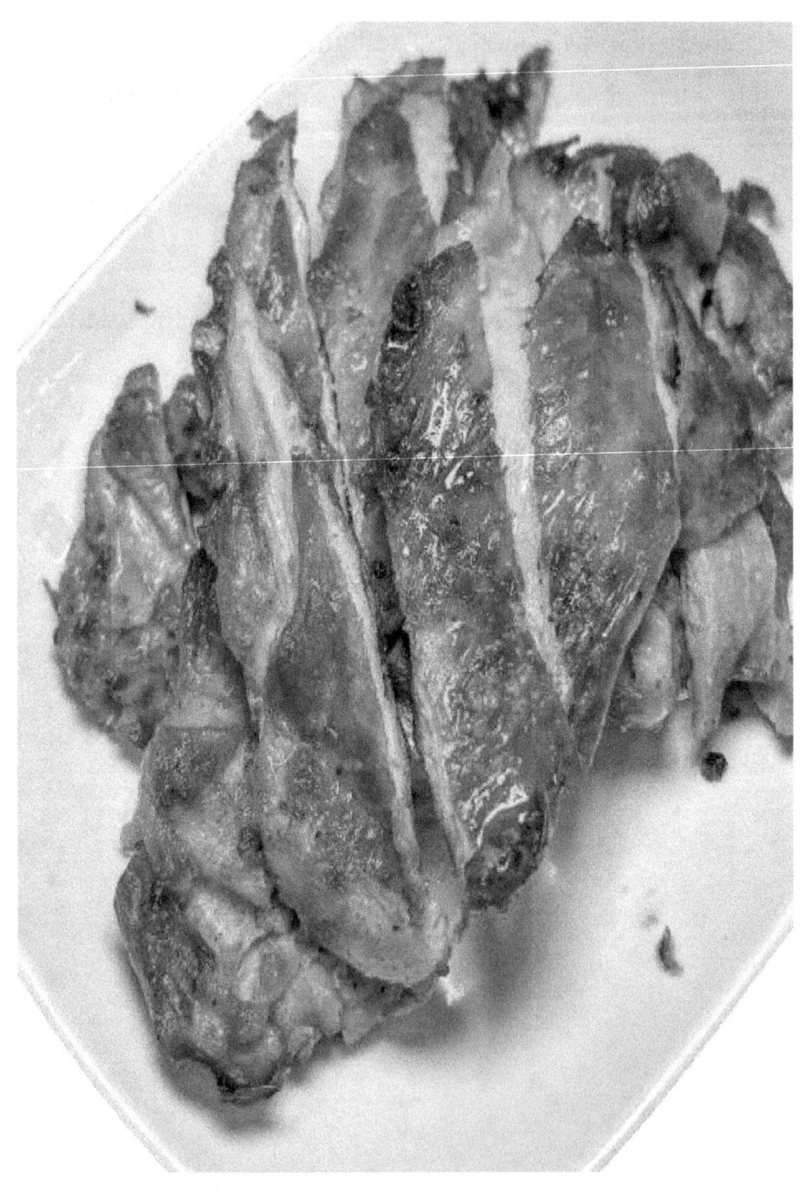

CONCLUSION

In conclusion, this book has been carefully crafted to provide flavorful and satisfying meals while adhering to heart-healthy guidelines.

The recipes included are not only delicious but also designed to support heart health and overall well-being.

By focusing on ingredients that are low in sodium, saturated fats, and cholesterol, and rich in fiber, vitamins, and minerals, this cookbook aims to help you with congestive heart failure manage your condition and improve your quality of life.

By incorporating these recipes into your daily routine, you can enjoy a variety of flavors and textures while taking care of your heart.

I hope that this cookbook has inspired you to explore new ingredients and cooking techniques, and that it has helped you to make healthier choices for yourself and your loved ones. Remember, eating well is not just about nourishing your body, but also about feeding your soul. Here's to good health and delicious meals!

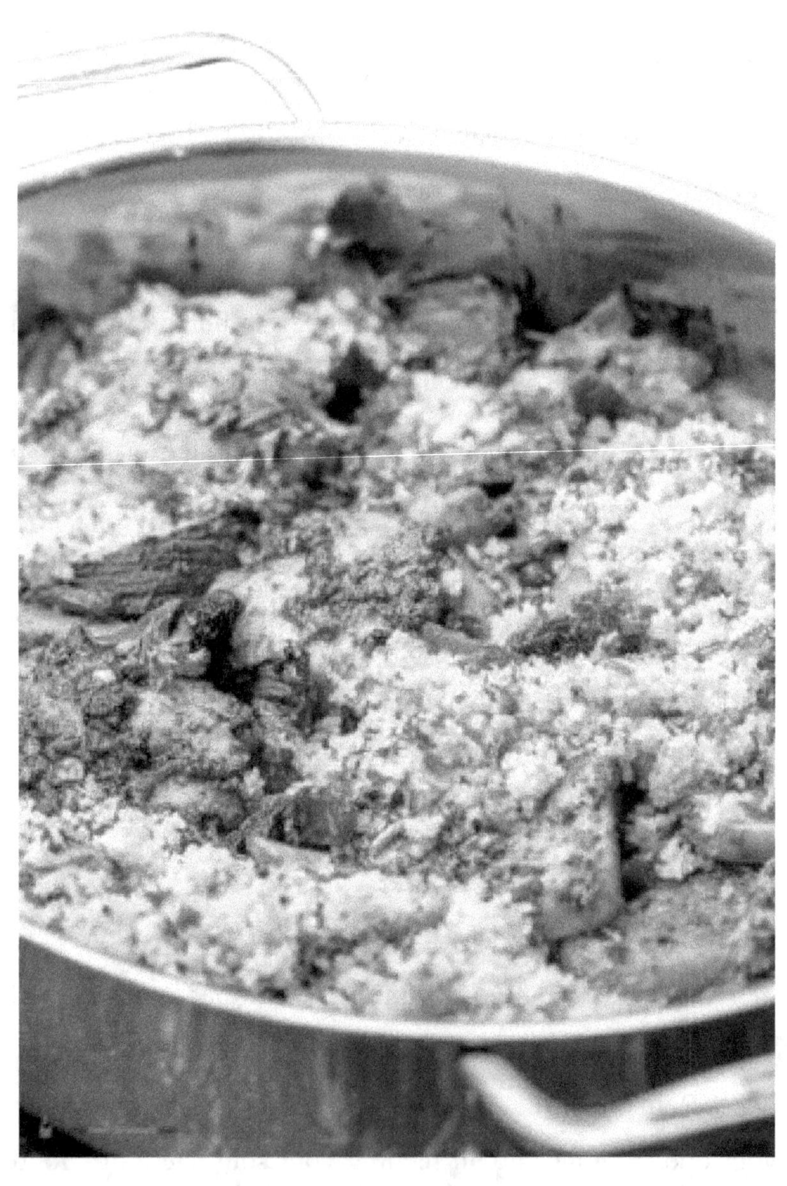